# Healthy aging and senior fitness

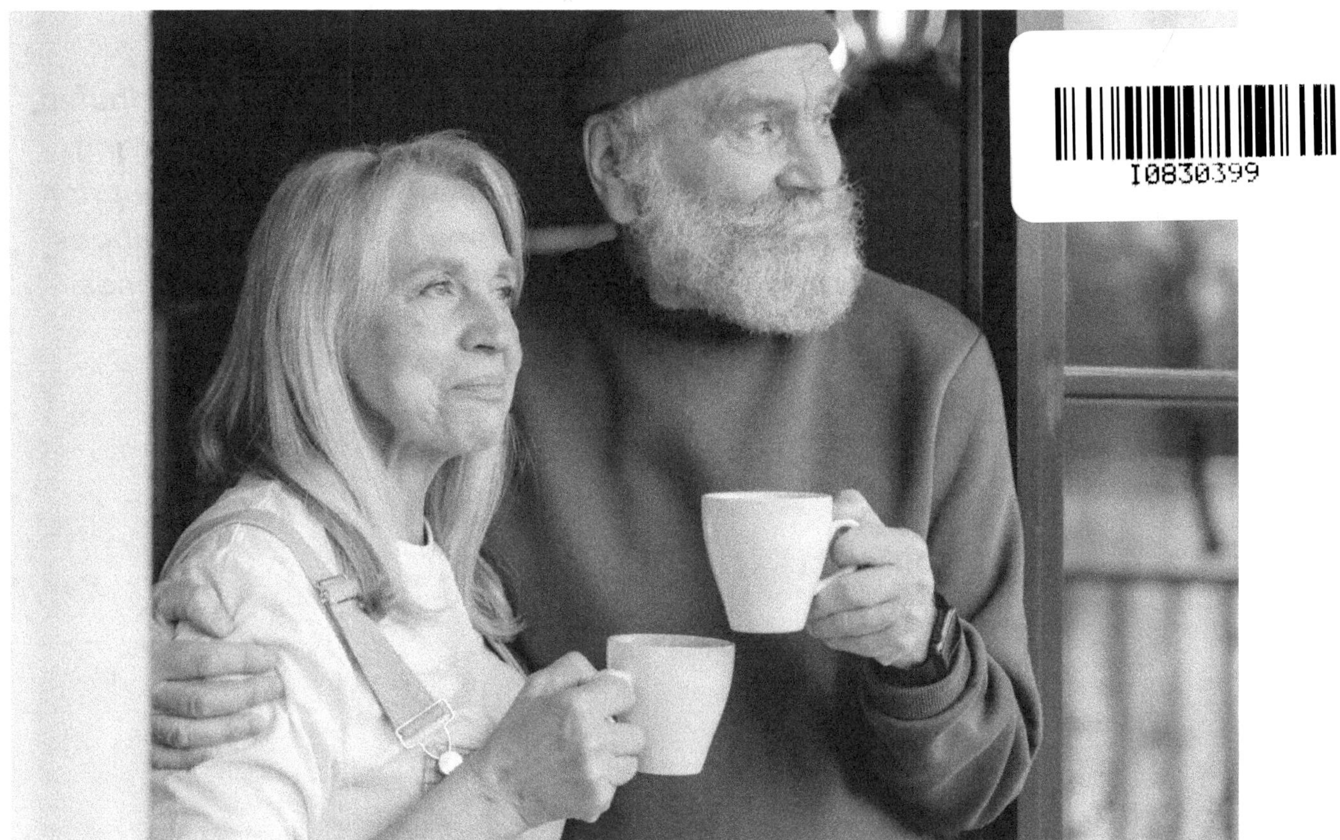

*Address the unique needs of older adults, including exercises to improve mobility, prevent falls, and maintain overall health.*

Copyright © [2023]
[HARRIS SMITH]

All rights reserved. No part of this ebook may be reproduced, distributed, or transmitted in any form or by any means, including photocopying, recording, or other electronic or mechanical methods, without the prior written permission of the author, except in the case of brief quotations embodied in critical reviews and certain other noncommercial uses permitted by copyright law.

Table of Contents

**Introduction**

# I. Introduction

A. Importance of healthy aging and senior fitness

B. Addressing the unique needs of older adults

# II. Chapter 1:

## Understanding Aging and Its Effects on the Body

A. The aging process and its impact on mobility and overall health

B. Common age-related conditions and their   effects

C. Importance of exercise for healthy aging

# III. Chapter 2:

## Assessing Individual Needs and Abilities

A. Evaluating physical capabilities and limitations

B. Identifying specific health concerns and risks

C. Tailoring exercise programs to individual needs

# IV. Chapter 3:

## Mobility and Flexibility Exercises

A. Importance of maintaining mobility and flexibility in older adults

B. Gentle stretching exercises to improve flexibility

C. Range-of-motion exercises to enhance joint mobility

# V. Chapter 4:

## Strength Training for Seniors

A. Benefits of strength training for older adults

B. Safe and effective strength exercises using bodyweight and resistance bands

# Introduction:

*Welcome to "Healthy Aging and Senior Fitness: Addressing the Unique Needs of Older Adults." In this book, we embark on a journey to explore the crucial elements of maintaining physical well-being, mobility, and overall health as we age gracefully. The aging process is an inevitable part of life, and it presents us with unique challenges and opportunities. By understanding and addressing these needs, we can embrace the joys of healthy aging and optimize our senior years.*

*A. Importance of Healthy Aging and Senior Fitness: In recent years, there has been a growing realization of the importance of healthy aging and senior fitness. With advancements in healthcare and improved lifestyles, people are living longer than ever before. However, the goal is not merely to extend our lifespan, but to ensure that these additional years are filled with vitality, independence, and a high quality of life.*

*Engaging in regular exercise and adopting a healthy lifestyle are crucial components of achieving this goal. Physical activity has been proven to enhance cardiovascular health, strengthen bones and muscles, improve cognitive function, and boost overall well-being. By embracing fitness as a lifelong journey, we can mitigate the risks of chronic diseases and maintain our physical and mental capabilities well into our senior years.*

*B. Addressing the Unique Needs of Older Adults: Aging brings about changes in our bodies and minds that require specific attention and care. As we advance in age, our muscles lose strength, bones become more fragile, and flexibility diminishes. Additionally, cognitive abilities may decline, and chronic conditions such as arthritis, diabetes, or heart disease may emerge. It is essential to address these unique needs through tailored exercises, modifications, and lifestyle adjustments.*

*This book aims to provide a comprehensive guide for older adults, their families, and fitness professionals who work with seniors. It offers a wealth of knowledge and practical advice on exercises specifically designed to improve mobility, prevent falls, and maintain overall health. We will delve into various forms of physical activity, including strength training, balance exercises, flexibility routines, cardiovascular workouts, and mindful movement practices. Alongside the exercises, we will explore nutrition tips, stress management techniques, and strategies for enhancing cognitive function.*

*By taking a holistic approach to senior fitness, we can unlock the immense potential that lies within us, regardless of age. It is never too late to invest in our well-being and embrace the transformative power of a healthy lifestyle. Together, let us embark on this empowering journey towards healthy aging, embracing vitality, and living life to the fullest.*

*Join me as we discover the secrets to maintaining optimal physical and mental health, ensuring that our golden years are filled with strength, joy, and the freedom to enjoy all that life has to offer.*

# Chapter 1:
## Understanding Aging and Its     Effects on the Body

### A. The Aging Process and Its Impact on Mobility and Overall Health

*Aging is a natural and inevitable process that affects every individual. As we grow older, our bodies undergo various physiological changes that can impact our mobility and overall health. Understanding the aging process is essential for addressing the unique needs of older adults and promoting healthy aging.*

*The aging process affects different systems in our body, including musculoskeletal, cardiovascular, neurological, and metabolic systems. These changes can lead to a decline in physical function, which may affect mobility, balance, strength, and flexibility.*

*Musculoskeletal changes often involve a loss of muscle mass and strength, known as sarcopenia, as well as a decrease in bone density, leading to osteoporosis. These changes can result in decreased mobility, increased frailty, and a higher risk of falls and fractures.*

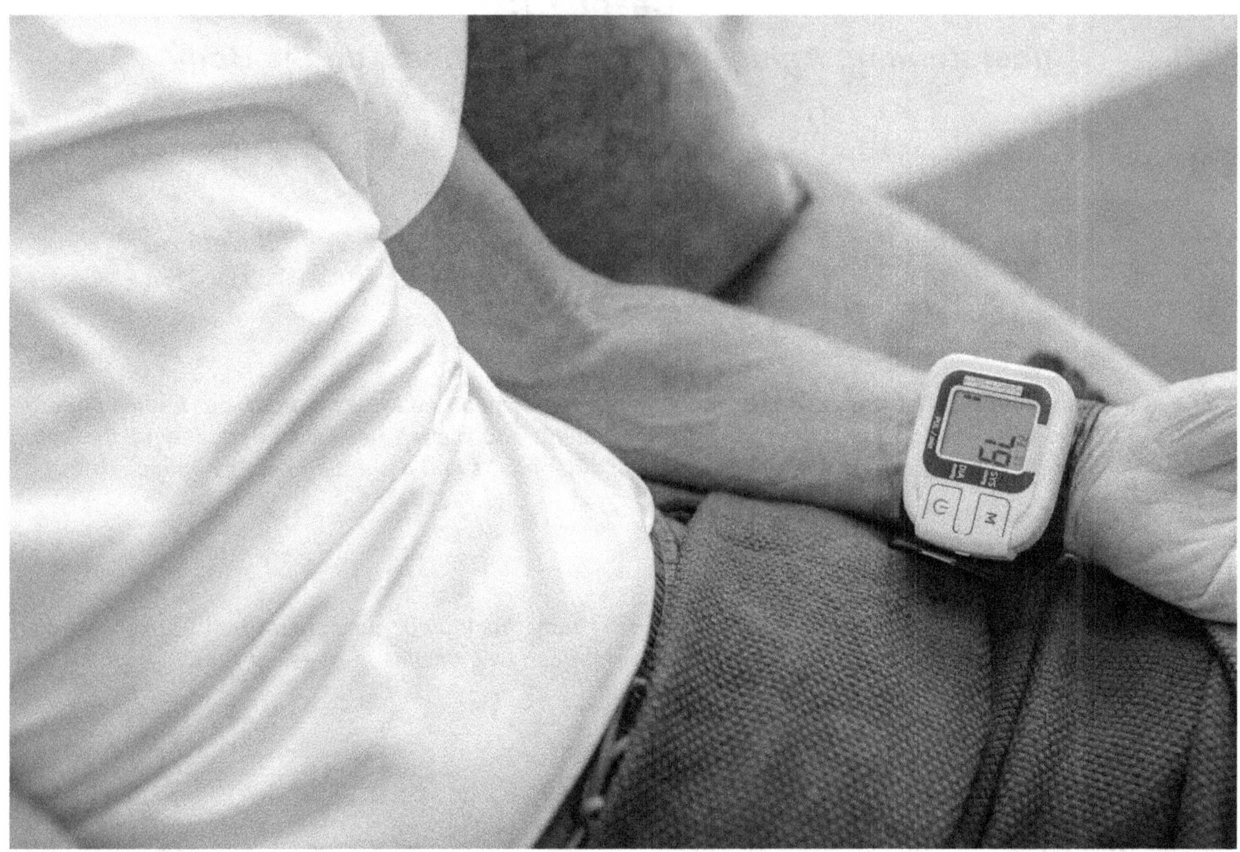

*Cardiovascular changes can include decreased cardiac output, reduced elasticity of blood vessels, and increased blood pressure. These alterations can contribute to decreased endurance, reduced ability to perform physical activities, and an increased risk of cardiovascular diseases.*

*Neurological changes may affect cognitive function, coordination, and balance. These changes can lead to decreased motor control and an increased risk of falls.*

*Metabolic changes involve a decrease in metabolic rate and changes in body composition, such as an increase in body fat and a decrease in lean muscle mass. These changes can affect overall energy levels, metabolism, and the body's ability to maintain a healthy weight.*

## B. Common Age-Related Conditions and Their Effects

*Alongside the natural aging process, older adults are more susceptible to developing age-related conditions that can further impact mobility and overall health. These conditions can include arthritis, osteoporosis, cardiovascular diseases, diabetes, and cognitive decline.*

*Arthritis is a common condition characterized by joint inflammation, pain, and stiffness. It can limit mobility and make movement challenging, affecting daily activities and quality of life.*

*Osteoporosis is a condition in which bones become weak and brittle, increasing the risk of fractures. It can lead to significant limitations in mobility and independence.*

*Cardiovascular diseases, such as heart disease and stroke, become more prevalent with age. These conditions can impair cardiovascular function, leading to reduced endurance, fatigue, and a higher risk of other health complications.*

*Diabetes is a metabolic disorder characterized by high blood sugar levels. It can lead to complications such as neuropathy and poor circulation, affecting mobility and overall health.*

*Cognitive decline, including conditions like Alzheimer's disease, can impact memory, thinking abilities, and overall cognitive function. These changes can affect mobility, balance, and safety.*

## C.Importance of Exercise for Healthy Aging

*Despite the challenges posed by the aging process and age-related conditions, there is strong evidence to support the importance of exercise for healthy aging. Engaging in regular physical activity has numerous benefits for older adults, both physically and mentally.*

*Exercise plays a pivotal role in maintaining and improving mobility, strength, flexibility, and balance. By incorporating exercises that target these areas, older adults can enhance their functional abilities, reduce the risk of falls, and maintain independence in performing daily tasks.*

*Regular physical activity also improves cardiovascular health, lowering the risk of heart disease, stroke, and high blood pressure. It enhances circulation, strengthens the heart muscle, and improves overall cardiovascular fitness.*

*Exercise has a positive impact on mental health as well. It reduces the risk of depression and anxiety, improves cognitive function, and enhances overall well-being. Physical activity stimulates the release of endorphins, which are natural mood-boosting chemicals in the brain.*

*Additionally, exercise promotes healthy weight management, improves bone density, and enhances metabolism. It can also reduce the risk of developing chronic conditions such as diabetes and certain types of cancer.*

*In the following chapters, we will explore.*

# Chapter 2:
## Assessing Individual Needs and Abilities

### A. Evaluating Physical Capabilities and Limitations

*Before embarking on a senior fitness program, it is crucial to evaluate the individual's physical capabilities and limitations. This assessment serves as the foundation for tailoring exercise programs to meet the unique needs of older adults.*

*Physical capabilities encompass factors such as strength, flexibility, balance, cardiovascular endurance, and coordination. Assessing these aspects provides insights into the starting point and progressions that can be incorporated into the exercise regimen.*

*Functional fitness assessments are valuable tools for evaluating physical capabilities. These assessments involve measuring an individual's ability to perform everyday tasks, such as walking, climbing stairs, reaching, and balancing. Additionally, strength tests, such as grip strength measurements and lower body strength assessments, provide valuable information about overall physical fitness.*

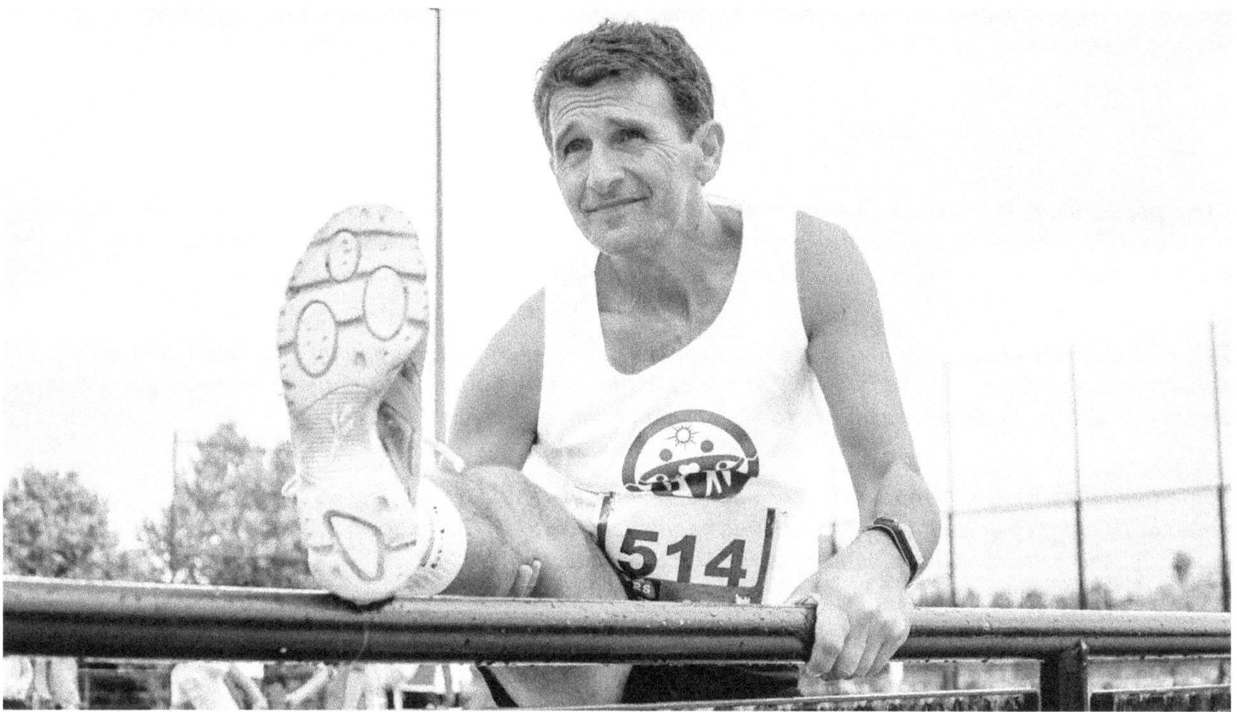

*Flexibility and range of motion assessments help identify any limitations or areas that require attention. By evaluating balance and stability, we can pinpoint potential fall risks and develop targeted exercises to improve stability and prevent falls.*

## B. Identifying Specific Health Concerns and Risks

*In addition to evaluating physical capabilities, it is essential to identify specific health concerns and risks that may impact exercise programs for older adults. Understanding these factors allows for the customization of exercise routines to ensure they are safe and effective.*

*Health concerns may include chronic conditions such as arthritis, heart disease, diabetes, or respiratory issues. These conditions may require modifications to exercise intensity, duration, or specific movements to accommodate individual needs. Consulting with healthcare professionals and considering any medical recommendations is crucial when designing exercise programs.*

*Identifying fall risks is another critical aspect. Falls are a significant concern for older adults, as they can lead to severe injuries and impact overall mobility and independence. Factors contributing to fall risks include muscle weakness, balance issues, medication side effects, and environmental hazards. By recognizing these risks, we can incorporate balance exercises and fall prevention strategies into exercise programs.*

## C. Tailoring Exercise Programs to Individual Needs

*Once physical capabilities, limitations, health concerns, and risks have been assessed, the next step is to tailor exercise programs to meet the individual needs of older adults. A personalized approach ensures that exercises are safe, effective, and enjoyable while addressing specific goals and concerns.*

*Tailoring an exercise program involves selecting appropriate exercises, modifying intensity and duration, and considering any necessary adaptations. It may also include incorporating equipment, such as resistance bands, stability balls, or chair support, to assist with certain exercises.*

*For individuals with limited mobility or chronic conditions, low-impact exercises such as water aerobics, gentle yoga, or tai chi may be suitable options. These activities provide benefits for cardiovascular health, strength, flexibility, and balance while minimizing stress on the joints.*

*Strength training exercises should focus on functional movements that improve overall muscle strength and enhance everyday activities. Balance exercises can help improve stability and reduce the risk of falls. Flexibility routines should target specific areas of concern, such as tight muscles or limited range of motion.*

*Regular reassessment is crucial to monitor progress, adjust exercise programs, and accommodate any changes in physical capabilities or health status. This ongoing evaluation ensures that exercise routines remain relevant and effective throughout the aging process.*

*By tailoring exercise programs to individual needs, we can maximize the benefits of physical activity while minimizing the risk of injury or overexertion. It is important to approach exercise as a personalized journey that promotes overall health, mobility, and well-being for older adults.*

*In the next chapter, we will delve into specific exercises and strategies designed to improve mobility, prevent falls, and maintain overall health. These exercises will encompass a range of activities suitable for different abilities and interests. Together, let us embrace the power of tailored exercise programs to support healthy aging and ensure a vibrant, active lifestyle for older adults.*

# *Chapter 3:*
# *Mobility and Flexibility Exercises*

## *A. Importance of Maintaining Mobility and Flexibility in Older Adults*

*Maintaining mobility and flexibility is crucial for older adults to enhance their overall health and quality of life. As we age, our bodies naturally experience a decrease in flexibility and mobility due to factors such as decreased activity levels, loss of muscle mass, and changes in joint structure. However, incorporating regular mobility and flexibility exercises can counteract these effects and help older adults maintain their independence and functional abilities.*

*Mobility refers to the ability to move freely and easily, while flexibility refers to the range of motion in our joints and muscles. By focusing on improving both aspects, older adults can experience numerous benefits, including:*

*Enhanced Joint Health: Regular mobility and flexibility exercises help lubricate the joints, improve blood circulation, and maintain the health of cartilage and connective tissues. This can alleviate joint stiffness and reduce the risk of conditions such as arthritis.*

*Improved Balance and Stability: Mobility exercises that target balance and coordination can enhance stability and reduce the risk of falls. Flexibility exercises contribute to improved posture and body alignment, further supporting balance and stability.*

*Increased Independence: By maintaining mobility and flexibility, older adults can perform daily activities with greater ease and independence. Whether it's getting up from a chair, reaching overhead, or bending down to tie shoelaces, having optimal mobility and flexibility allows for greater functional independence.*

*Enhanced Performance in Physical Activities: Whether it's walking, gardening, or playing with grandchildren, maintaining mobility and flexibility ensures that older adults can participate in and enjoy various physical activities without discomfort or limitations.*

## *B. Gentle Stretching Exercises to Improve Flexibility*

*Flexibility exercises play a vital role in improving range of motion, reducing muscle tension, and preventing injuries. Incorporating gentle stretching exercises into a senior fitness routine can help improve flexibility and promote overall well-being. Some examples of gentle stretching exercises suitable for older adults include:*

*Neck Stretches: Gently tilt the head to the right and hold for 10-15 seconds, then repeat on the left side. Perform chin tucks by bringing the chin toward the chest to stretch the back of the neck.*

*Shoulder Rolls: Roll the shoulders forward and backward in a circular motion to release tension and improve mobility in the shoulder joints.*

*Chest Stretch: Stand upright, clasp your hands behind your back, and gently lift your arms away from your body to stretch the chest muscles.*

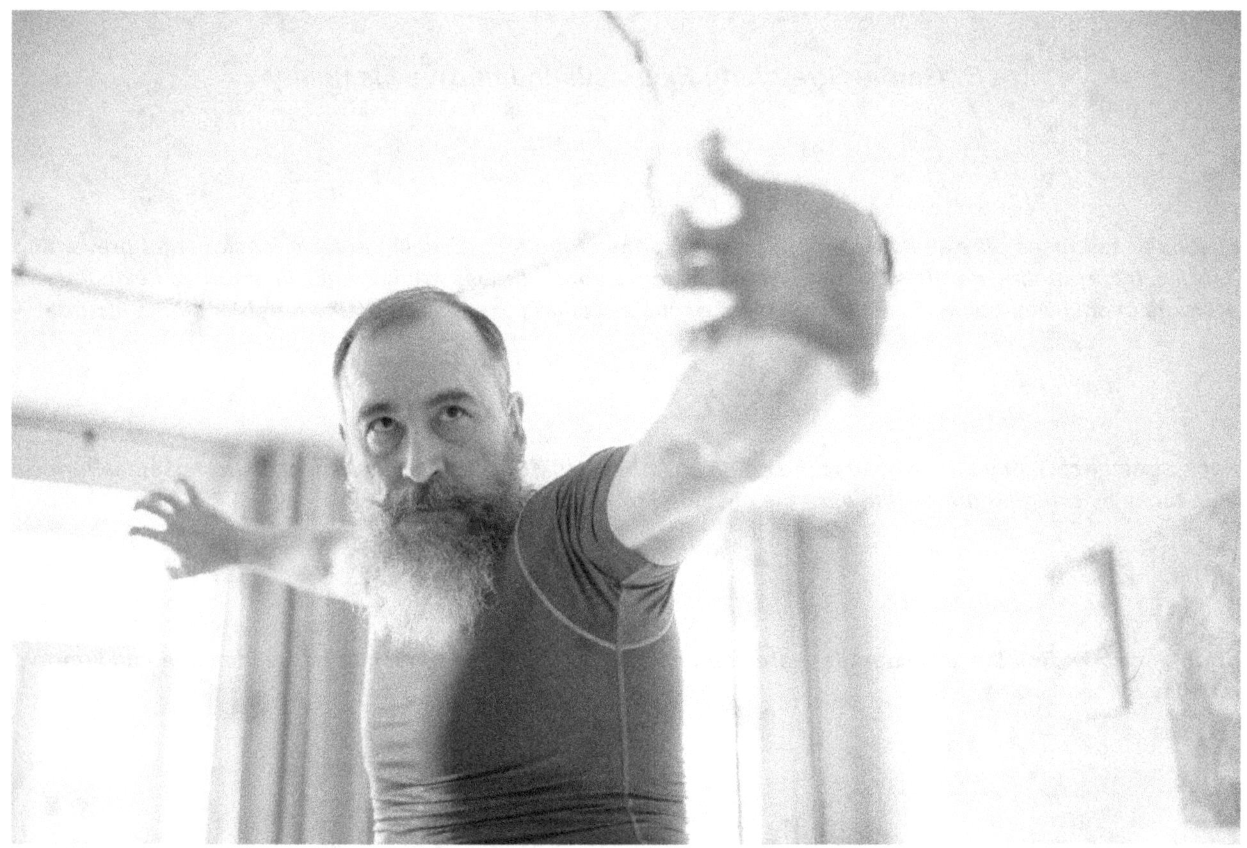

*Hamstring Stretches: Sit on the edge of a chair, extend one leg forward, and gently lean forward from the hips until you feel a gentle stretch in the back of the thigh. Hold for 10-15 seconds and repeat on the other leg.*

*Calf Stretches: Stand facing a wall, place your hands on the wall for support, and step one foot back while keeping the heel on the ground. Lean forward until you feel a stretch in the calf of the back leg. Hold for 10-15 seconds and repeat on the other leg.*

### *C. Range-of-Motion Exercises to Enhance Joint Mobility*

*Range-of-motion exercises focus on moving joints through their full range of motion to improve mobility and prevent stiffness. These exercises can help maintain joint flexibility and function. Here are some examples of range-of-motion exercises for different joints:*

*Shoulder Circles: Stand or sit with arms relaxed at your sides. Slowly raise both shoulders up towards the ears, roll them back, down, and forward in a smooth circular motion. Repeat 5-10 times.*

*Wrist Flexion and Extension: Extend one arm in front of you with the palm facing down. Use the other hand to gently bend the wrist upward, feeling a stretch in the forearm.*

# Chapter 4:
## Strength Training for Seniors

### A. Benefits of Strength Training for Older Adults

*Strength training, also known as resistance training or weightlifting, offers numerous benefits for older adults. It is a valuable component of a comprehensive fitness program, promoting healthy aging and supporting overall well-being. Here are some key benefits of strength training for seniors:*

*Increased Muscle Strength and Endurance: Strength training helps build and maintain muscle mass, which naturally declines with age. By engaging in regular resistance exercises, older adults can improve their muscle strength, allowing them to perform daily activities with greater ease and independence.*

*Enhanced Bone Health: Strength training helps increase bone density and reduce the risk of osteoporosis and fractures. By putting stress on the bones through resistance exercises, older adults can stimulate bone growth and maintain strong, healthy bones.*

*Improved Joint Health: Strengthening the muscles around the joints provides added support and stability, reducing the risk of joint pain and injuries. Strong muscles help alleviate pressure on the joints, enhancing joint function and mobility.*

*Enhanced Metabolism and Weight Management: Strength training increases lean muscle mass, which can boost the metabolism and help older adults maintain a healthy weight. As muscle tissue is more metabolically active than fat tissue, it can lead to increased calorie burn even at rest.*

*Improved Balance and Fall Prevention: Strength training exercises that target the lower body, such as squats and lunges, can improve balance and stability. This reduces the risk of falls and related injuries, promoting independence and confidence in daily activities.*

### *B. Safe and Effective Strength Exercises Using Bodyweight and Resistance Bands*

*Strength training for seniors can be safe, effective, and enjoyable, even without the use of heavy weights or gym equipment. Bodyweight exercises and resistance bands provide excellent alternatives that allow older adults to build strength and gain the benefits of strength training. Here are some safe and effective exercises:*

*Squats: Stand with feet shoulder-width apart, and slowly lower your body as if sitting back into a chair, keeping your knees aligned with your toes. Rise back up to the starting position. This exercise strengthens the leg muscles, including the quadriceps and glutes.*

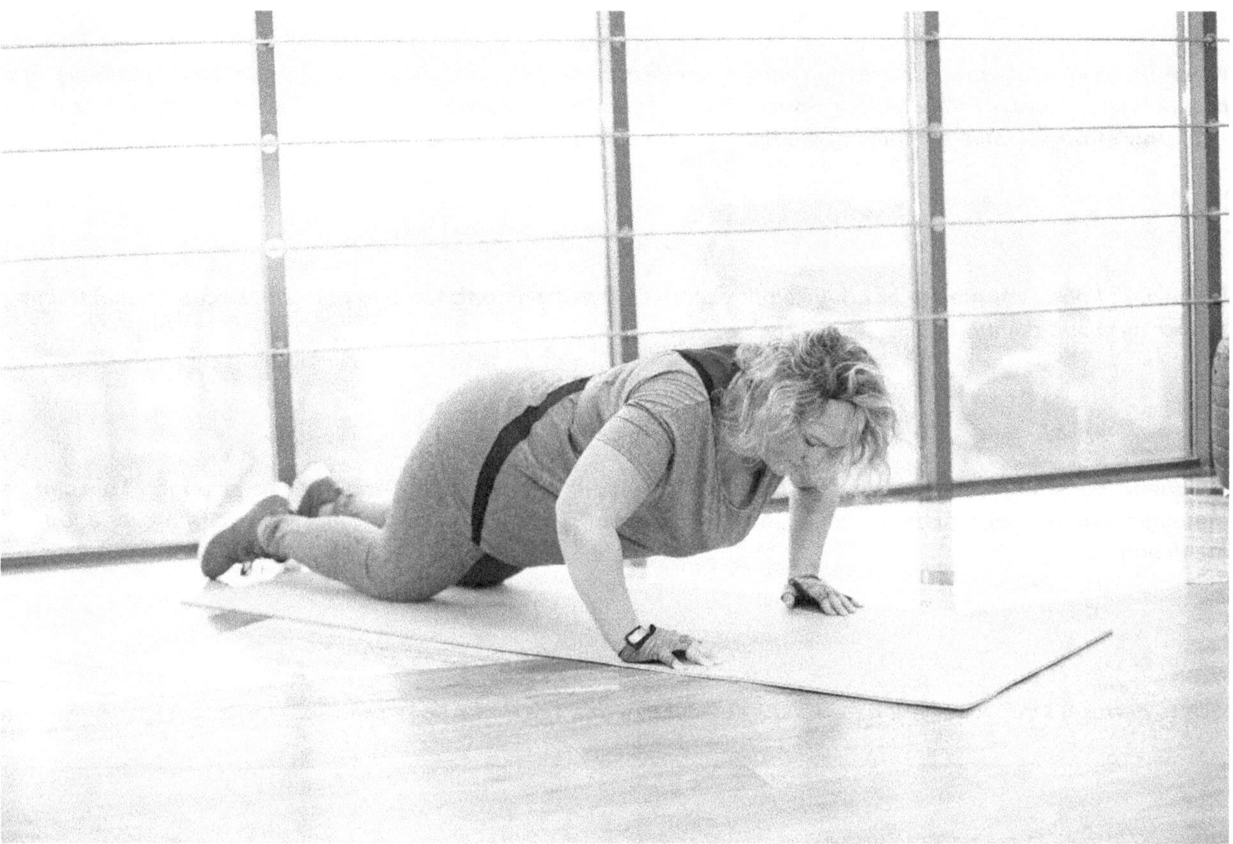

*Push-ups against a Wall or Elevated Surface: Stand facing a wall or use a stable surface like a countertop. Place your hands shoulder-width apart on the surface, and step back until your body is at a slight angle. Lower your chest towards the wall or surface and push back up. This exercise targets the chest, shoulders, and triceps.*

*Resistance Band Rows: Sit on a chair with your legs extended in front of you. Loop a resistance band around your feet and hold the ends with your hands. Pull the band towards your body, squeezing your shoulder blades together. This exercise strengthens the upper back muscles.*

*Leg Press with Resistance Band: Sit on a chair with your feet shoulder-width apart. Loop a resistance band around your feet and hold the ends. Push your feet forward against the resistance of the band, extending your knees. This exercise targets the quadriceps and glutes.*

## C. Progressive Resistance Training to Build Strength Gradually

*When incorporating strength training into a senior fitness program, it is important to start gradually and progressively increase the challenge over time. Progressive resistance training allows the muscles to adapt and grow stronger while minimizing the risk of injury. Here are some tips for progressive resistance training:*

*Begin with lighter resistance or bodyweight exercises that are comfortable to perform. Focus on maintaining proper form and technique.*

*Gradually increase the resistance or difficulty level as your muscles adapt and become stronger. This can be done by using thicker resistance bands, adding repetitions, or progressing to more challenging variations of the exercises.*

*Aim to perform strength training exercises at least two to three times per week.*

# Chapter 5:
## Cardiovascular Health and Aerobic Exercises

### A. Understanding the Importance of Cardiovascular Health for Seniors

*Maintaining cardiovascular health is vital for seniors to enhance their overall well-being and quality of life. Regular aerobic exercise, also known as cardio exercise, offers numerous benefits for older adults. It strengthens the heart, improves lung function, increases endurance, and helps manage weight. Furthermore, cardiovascular exercise can reduce the risk of chronic diseases such as heart disease, high blood pressure, diabetes, and stroke. By prioritizing cardiovascular health, older adults can enjoy increased energy levels, improved mood, and a decreased risk of age-related decline.*

### B. Low-Impact Aerobic Exercises for Older Adults

*When it comes to aerobic exercises for older adults, low-impact activities are particularly beneficial. These exercises are gentle on the joints, reduce the risk of injury, and can be easily modified to accommodate different fitness levels. Here are some low-impact aerobic exercises suitable for seniors:*

*Walking: Walking is a simple and accessible exercise that can be done indoors or outdoors. Start with shorter distances and gradually increase the duration and pace. Consider walking in nature, at a local park, or with a walking group to make it more enjoyable.*

*Cycling: Whether on a stationary bike or outdoors, cycling provides a low-impact cardiovascular workout. Adjust the resistance or incline to challenge yourself and improve endurance. Consider group cycling classes or cycling on scenic paths to add variety to your routine.*

*Swimming: Swimming is a fantastic low-impact exercise that provides a full-body workout. It is gentle on the joints and offers resistance, strengthening muscles and improving cardiovascular fitness. Try water aerobics or aqua jogging for additional variety.*

*Dancing: Dancing is not only a fun and social activity but also an excellent aerobic exercise. Whether taking dance classes or simply dancing at home, it improves cardiovascular fitness, coordination, and balance.*

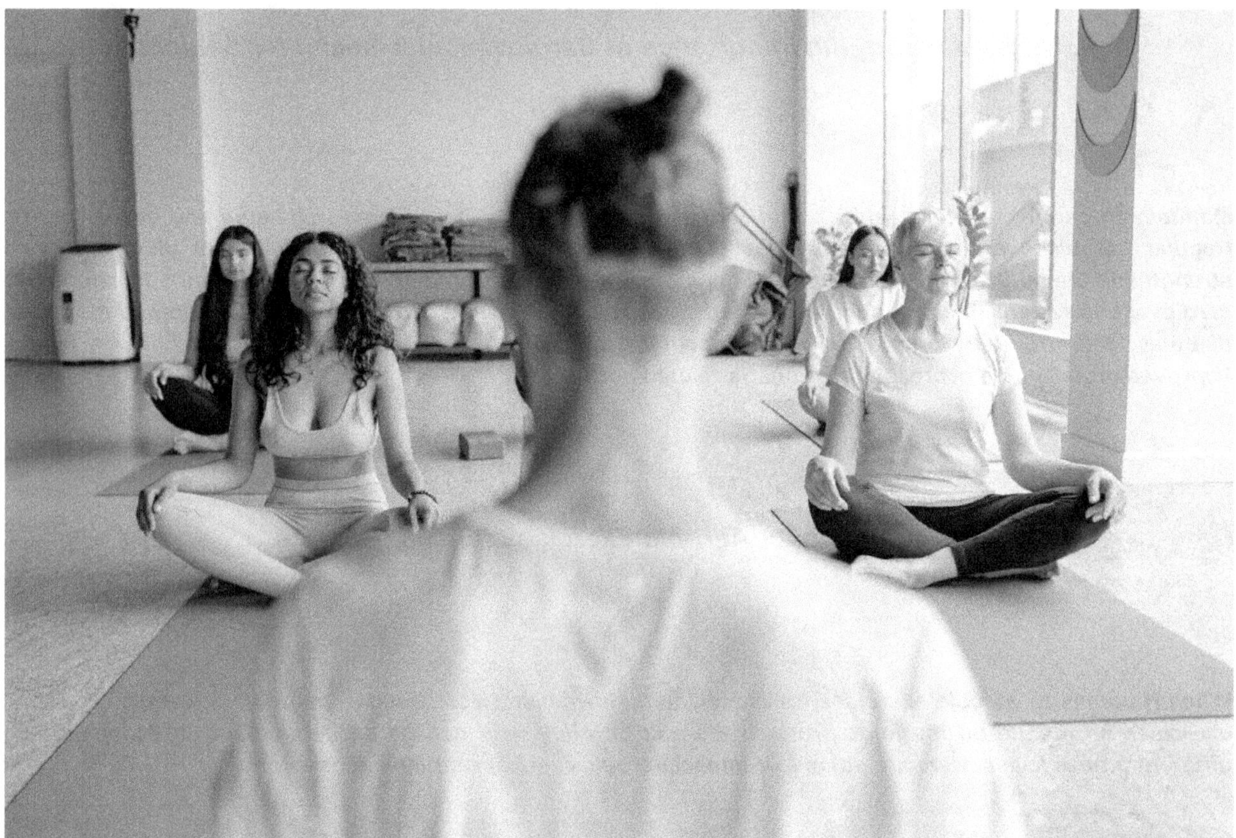

*Tai Chi: Tai Chi combines gentle movements with deep breathing, promoting relaxation and cardiovascular fitness. It focuses on balance, flexibility, and mind-body connection, making it suitable for older adults of all fitness levels.*

## *C. Incorporating Cardiovascular Activities into Daily Routines*

*In addition to dedicated aerobic exercises, it is essential to incorporate cardiovascular activities into daily routines. Making small lifestyle changes can have a significant impact on cardiovascular health. Here are some practical ways to increase daily activity levels:*

*Take the stairs instead of the elevator or escalator whenever possible. Climbing stairs engages the leg muscles and increases heart rate, providing a cardiovascular workout.*

*Choose active transportation options such as walking or cycling for short distances instead of relying solely on cars or public transportation.*

*Engage in household chores and gardening activities that involve continuous movement, such as vacuuming, mowing the lawn, or raking leaves.*

*Break up sedentary periods by incorporating regular movement breaks. Take short walks, do light stretching, or perform simple exercises like marching in place or chair squats.*

*Participate in group fitness classes or community programs specifically designed for seniors. These classes often include low-impact aerobic exercises, providing an opportunity for social interaction and motivation.*

*Remember to consult with a healthcare professional before starting any new exercise program, especially if you have pre-existing health conditions. They can provide personalized guidance and ensure that aerobic exercises are safe and suitable for your individual needs.*

*By prioritizing cardiovascular health and incorporating low-impact aerobic exercises into daily routines, older adults can enjoy improved cardiovascular fitness, increased energy levels, and a reduced risk of age-related health conditions. Embrace the joy of movement and strive for a heart-healthy lifestyle to support healthy aging and overall well-being.*

## *A. Addressing the Risks of Falls in Older Adults*

*Falls are a significant concern for older adults, as they can lead to serious injuries, decreased independence, and a decline in overall health. Understanding and addressing the risks associated with falls is crucial for maintaining the well-being of older adults. Factors that contribute to the risk of falls include muscle weakness, poor balance, impaired vision, medication side effects, and environmental hazards. By recognizing and addressing these risks, we can take proactive steps to prevent falls and promote safe, independent living for older adults.*

## *B.Exercises to Improve Balance and Stability*

*Improving balance and stability through targeted exercises is an effective way to reduce the risk of falls in older adults. These exercises focus on strengthening the core muscles, improving proprioception (the sense of body position in space), and enhancing overall body control. Here are some exercises that can help improve balance and stability:*

*Single-Leg Stance: Stand near a sturdy support, such as a chair, and lift one foot off the ground. Try to maintain your balance on the other leg for 20-30 seconds. Repeat on the other leg. As you become more confident, gradually increase the duration of the exercise.*

*Heel-to-Toe Walk: Position the heel of one foot directly in front of the toes of the opposite foot, as if walking on a tightrope. Take small steps in this manner for about 10-15 steps. This exercise challenges balance and coordination.*

*Standing Leg Swings: Stand near a wall or support and swing one leg forward and backward, like a pendulum. Start with small swings and gradually increase the range of motion. Repeat for 10-15 swings on each leg. This exercise helps improve dynamic balance.*

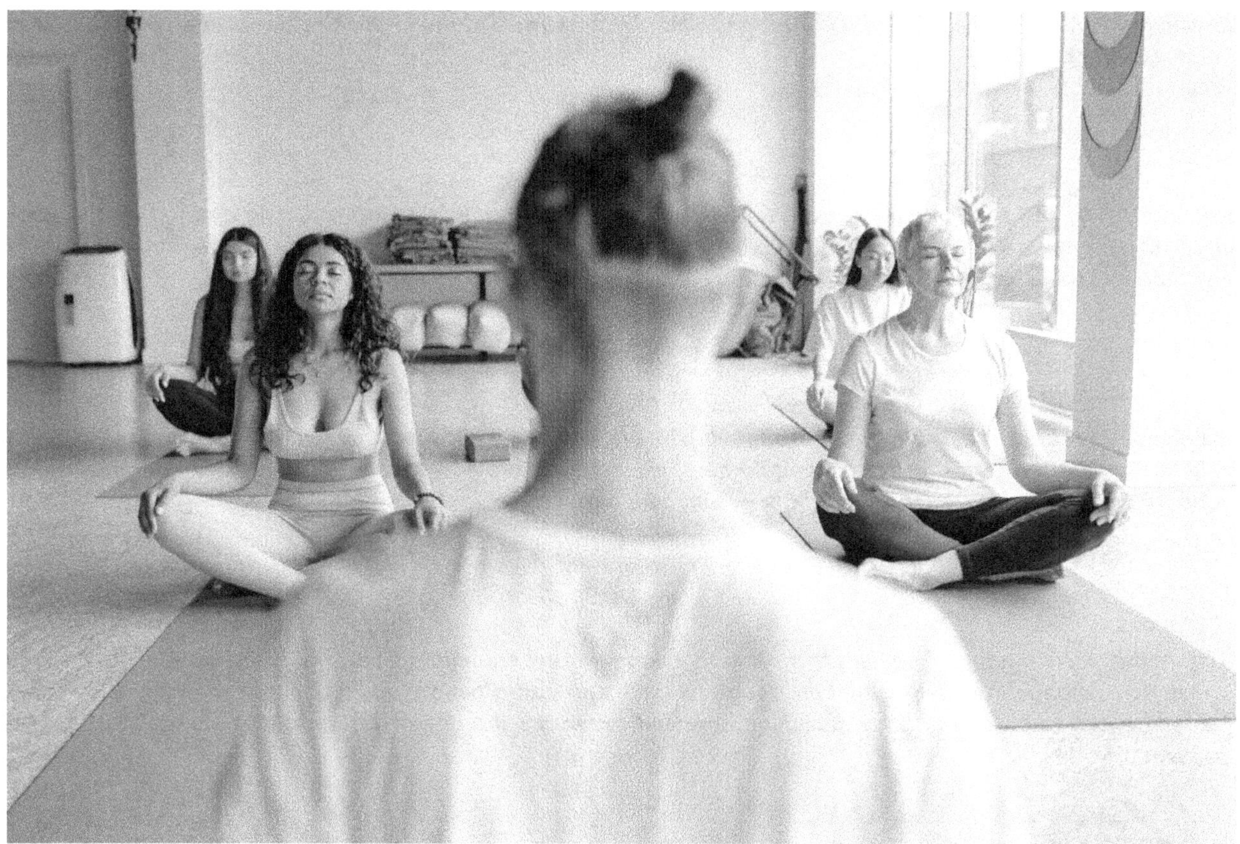

*Yoga or Tai Chi: Engaging in mind-body practices such as yoga or tai chi can significantly improve balance and stability. These practices focus on controlled movements, deep breathing, and body awareness, promoting both physical and mental well-being.*

### *C.Strategies for Fall Prevention and Creating a Safe Environment*

*In addition to exercises, implementing strategies for fall prevention and creating a safe environment is essential for older adults. Here are some key considerations:*

*Remove Hazards: Conduct a thorough assessment of the living environment and remove any potential hazards. Secure loose rugs, ensure adequate lighting, and keep pathways clear of clutter. Install handrails on stairs and in bathrooms to provide support and stability.*

*Use Assistive Devices: For individuals who may have balance issues, using assistive devices such as canes or walkers can provide additional support and stability. Ensure that these devices are properly fitted and in good working condition.*

*Regular Vision and Medication Checks: Schedule regular eye examinations to maintain optimal vision. Poor vision can increase the risk of falls. Additionally, review medications with a healthcare professional to identify any that may have side effects affecting balance or coordination.*

*Fall-Proof Your Exercise Routine: When engaging in exercise or physical activity, ensure that the environment is safe. Use sturdy chairs or exercise equipment, wear appropriate footwear with good traction, and have a support system in place, such as a spotter or exercise partner.*

*Stay Active and Engaged: Regular physical activity and mental stimulation are vital for overall health and fall prevention. Engage in activities that challenge balance and coordination, such as dance classes or balance-focused exercise programs. Stay socially connected to reduce the risk of isolation and maintain a positive mindset.*

*By combining targeted balance and stability exercises with fall prevention strategies and a safe environment, older adults can significantly reduce their risk of falls and maintain their independence. Remember, it's never too late to start working on balance and fall prevention. Empower yourself or your loved ones with the knowledge and tools to stay.*

# Chapter 7:
## Maintaining Cognitive Health and Mental Well-being

### A. Relationship between Physical Exercise and Cognitive Function

*Physical exercise not only benefits the body but also plays a significant role in maintaining cognitive health and promoting mental well-being in older adults. Research has shown a strong relationship between physical activity and cognitive function. Regular exercise improves blood flow to the brain, stimulates the growth of new neurons, and enhances the release of neurotransmitters that support cognitive function. It has been linked to improved memory, attention, and executive function, as well as a reduced risk of cognitive decline and dementia. By incorporating physical exercise into their daily routines, older adults can support their cognitive health and maintain mental sharpness.*

### B. Activities to Promote Mental Stimulation and Memory Retention.

*Engaging in activities that promote mental stimulation and memory retention is crucial for older adults to maintain cognitive health and mental well-being. Here are some activities that can be incorporated into daily life:*

*1.Brain Games and Puzzles: Solving puzzles, playing strategic games, and engaging in activities such as crosswords, Sudoku, or chess can challenge the mind, improve cognitive abilities, and enhance memory retention.*

*2.Learning New Skills: Pursuing new hobbies or learning a new language or musical instrument can stimulate the brain and promote neuroplasticity, which is the brain's ability to adapt and form new connections.*

*3.Reading and Writing: Reading books, newspapers, or magazines, as well as engaging in writing activities such as journaling or creative writing, can enhance cognitive function, vocabulary, and verbal fluency.*

4.Social Engagement: Maintaining social connections and engaging in meaningful social activities can support cognitive health. Interacting with others, participating in group discussions or clubs, and volunteering can stimulate the brain and improve overall well-being.

4.Digital Brain Training Apps: There are various smartphone applications and online platforms specifically designed to provide brain-training exercises and activities. These apps offer a convenient way to engage in cognitive stimulation and track progress.

## C. Managing Stress and Promoting Emotional Well-being in Older Adults

Managing stress and promoting emotional well-being are essential for overall mental health in older adults. Chronic stress can negatively impact cognitive function and increase the risk of mental health issues. Here are some strategies to manage stress and promote emotional well-being:

Practice Relaxation Techniques: Engage in relaxation techniques such as deep breathing exercises, meditation, mindfulness, or yoga. These practices can help reduce stress, improve focus, and promote a sense of calm.

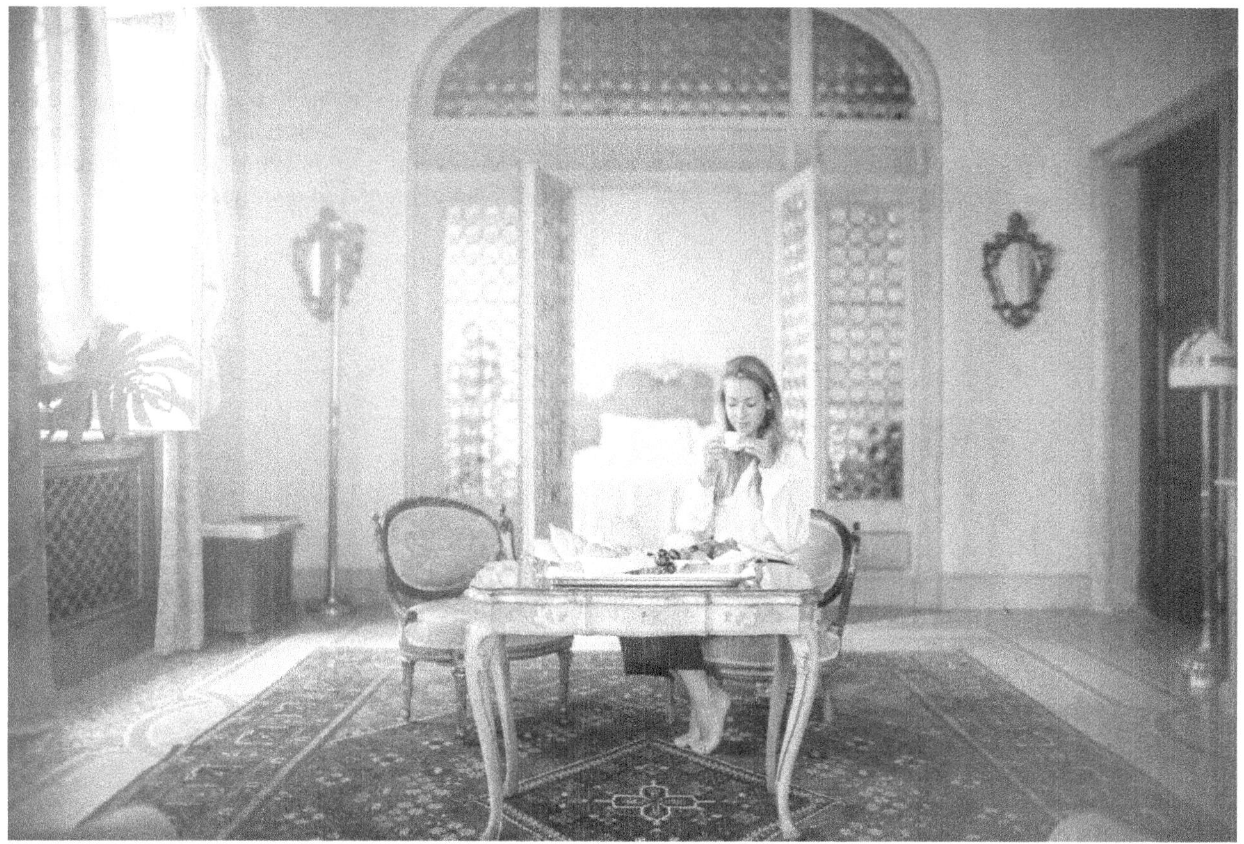

*Maintain a Healthy Lifestyle: A balanced diet, regular exercise, and sufficient sleep contribute to overall well-being and reduce the risk of stress and mental health issues. Establishing healthy habits supports emotional resilience and cognitive health.*

*Seek Emotional Support: Stay connected with family, friends, and support networks. Engage in meaningful conversations, share experiences, and seek emotional support when needed. Social interaction and a strong support system can provide comfort, reduce stress, and improve mental well-being.*

*Engage in Relaxing Activities: Find activities that bring joy and relaxation, such as listening to music, practicing hobbies, spending time in nature, or engaging in art therapy. These activities can promote emotional well-being and reduce stress levels.*

*Maintain a Positive Mindset: Cultivate a positive outlook by focusing on gratitude, practicing self-compassion, and engaging in positive self-talk. Embrace the power of optimism and resilience in dealing with life's challenges.*

*By incorporating physical exercise, engaging in mentally stimulating activities, and managing stress effectively, older adults can maintain cognitive health and promote mental well-being. These strategies contribute to a fulfilling and vibrant life, supporting healthy aging and overall quality of life. Remember to tailor these activities to individual preferences and capabilities, ensuring enjoyment and engagement.*

# Chapter 8:
## Nutrition and Healthy Eating Habits

### A. Importance of a Balanced Diet for Healthy Aging

*Maintaining a balanced diet is crucial for healthy aging and overall well-being in older adults. As we age, our bodies undergo various physiological changes that require specific nutrients to support optimal health. A balanced diet provides the necessary nutrients, vitamins, and minerals to promote healthy aging and prevent age-related diseases. It supports a strong immune system, maintains muscle mass and bone density, supports cognitive function, and helps manage chronic conditions such as diabetes, hypertension, and heart disease. By focusing on a balanced diet, older adults can improve their quality of life and enhance their overall health.*

### B. Nutritional Requirements and Considerations for Older Adults

*As we age, our nutritional requirements change, and it becomes essential to consider specific factors when planning a healthy diet. Here are some key considerations for older adults:*

*Adequate Protein Intake: Protein is crucial for maintaining muscle mass, promoting tissue repair, and supporting immune function. Older adults may need slightly higher protein intake to mitigate age-related muscle loss. Good sources of protein include lean meats, poultry, fish, eggs, dairy products, legumes, and nuts.*

*Increased Calcium and Vitamin D: Calcium and vitamin D are vital for maintaining bone health and preventing osteoporosis. Older adults may require higher amounts of these nutrients. Good sources of calcium include dairy products, leafy green vegetables, and fortified foods, while sunlight and fortified foods are essential sources of vitamin D.*

*Fiber-Rich Foods: Adequate fiber intake is crucial for maintaining digestive health, managing weight, and preventing constipation. Older adults should include a variety of fruits, vegetables, whole grains, legumes, and nuts in their diet to ensure sufficient fiber intake.*

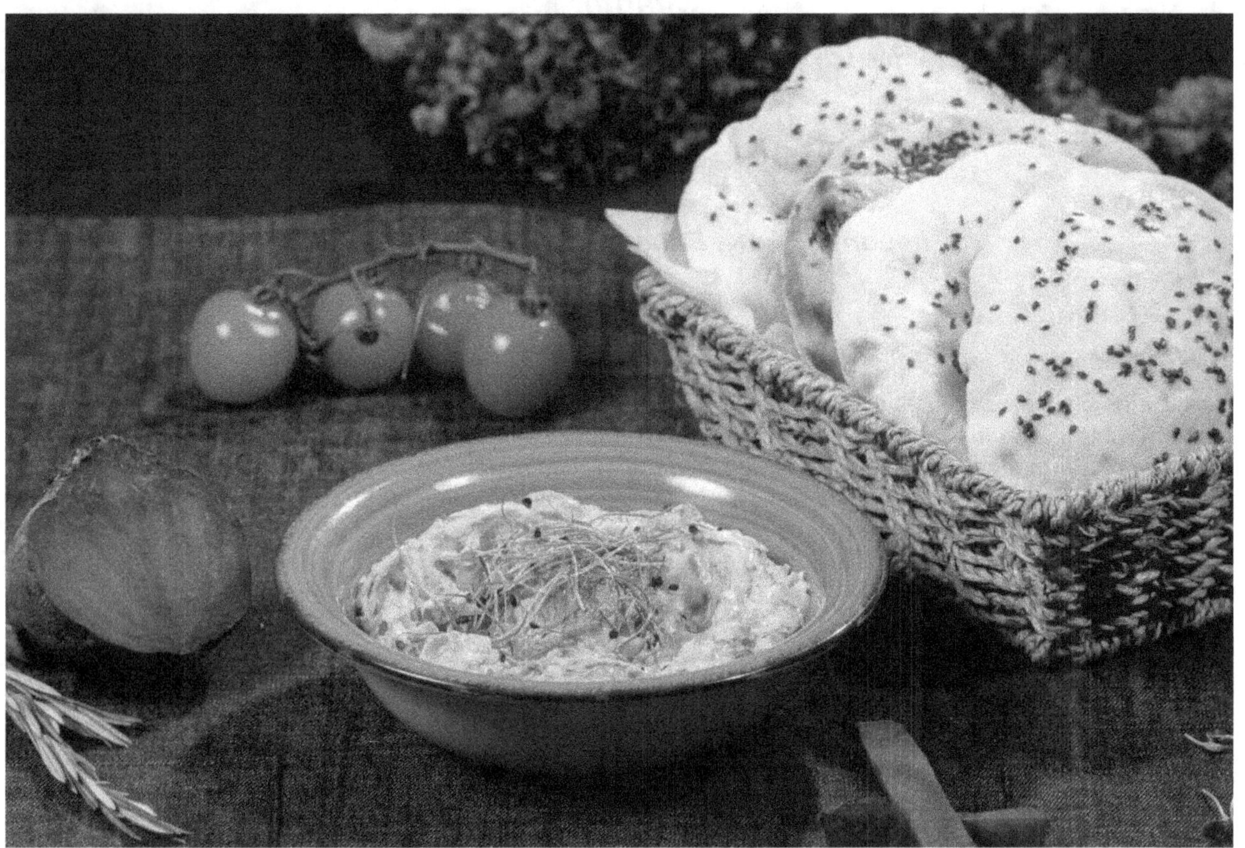

*Hydration: Older adults may be at a higher risk of dehydration due to decreased thirst sensation. It is important to maintain proper hydration by drinking water and consuming hydrating foods such as fruits, vegetables, and soups. Monitoring fluid intake is particularly important for those with certain medical conditions or taking medications that increase the risk of dehydration.*

*Micronutrients and Antioxidants: Ensuring an adequate intake of vitamins and minerals is crucial for supporting overall health and combating oxidative stress. Colorful fruits and vegetables, whole grains, nuts, seeds, and lean proteins are excellent sources of essential vitamins and minerals.*

### *C. Tips for Healthy Eating and Maintaining Proper Hydration*

*To maintain healthy eating habits and proper hydration, here are some practical tips for older adults:*

*Plan and Prepare Meals: Plan meals ahead of time to ensure a well-balanced diet. Include a variety of nutrient-dense foods and try new recipes to keep meals exciting and enjoyable. Consider meal prepping or cooking larger batches to have ready-made meals or leftovers for convenience.*

*Portion Control: Be mindful of portion sizes to avoid overeating. As metabolism slows down with age, portion control becomes important for maintaining a healthy weight and preventing overconsumption of calories.*

*Include a Variety of Foods: Aim to incorporate a variety of food groups in each meal to ensure a wide range of nutrients. Emphasize fruits, vegetables, whole grains, lean proteins, and healthy fats.*

*Limit Processed Foods and Added Sugars: Minimize the intake of processed foods, sugary snacks, and beverages. These foods provide little nutritional value and can contribute to weight gain and chronic health conditions.*

*Stay Active: Regular physical activity supports a healthy appetite and metabolism. Engaging in regular exercise can also help manage weight, improve digestion, and enhance overall well-being.*

*Seek Professional Advice: If you have specific dietary concerns or medical conditions, consult a registered dietitian or healthcare professional who specializes in nutrition. They can provide personalized advice.*

*Chapter 9:*
# *Creating an Active Lifestyle and Social Connections*

## *A. Promoting an Active Lifestyle beyond Structured Exercises*

*Maintaining an active lifestyle goes beyond structured exercise routines and plays a vital role in healthy aging for older adults. Engaging in regular physical activity not only improves physical health but also enhances mental well-being and overall quality of life. Here are some ways to promote an active lifestyle:*

*Daily Movement: Incorporate physical activity into daily routines by taking the stairs instead of the elevator, walking or cycling for short errands, or engaging in household chores that require movement. Small changes like these can add up and contribute to an active lifestyle.*

*Active Hobbies: Explore hobbies and activities that involve movement, such as gardening, dancing, swimming, golfing, or hiking. These activities not only provide exercise but also bring joy and fulfillment.*

*Outdoor Exploration: Take advantage of the natural environment and explore outdoor activities. Walking in nature, participating in community walks or group fitness classes, or joining local sports clubs can provide opportunities for physical activity while enjoying the outdoors.*

*Active Transportation: Opt for active modes of transportation whenever possible, such as walking or cycling. Not only does this contribute to physical activity, but it also helps reduce carbon footprint and supports environmental sustainability.*

## *B. Engaging in Social Activities and Maintaining Social Connections*

*Social connections play a significant role in healthy aging and overall well-being. Engaging in social activities and maintaining meaningful relationships can have a positive impact on mental and emotional health. Here are some ways to promote social connections:*

*Community Involvement: Participate in community activities, local clubs, or senior centers. These provide opportunities to meet like-minded individuals, engage in group activities, and contribute to the community.*

*Volunteering: Engaging in volunteer work allows older adults to make a difference in the lives of others while fostering social connections. It provides a sense of purpose, fulfillment, and the opportunity to meet people with shared interests.*

*Joining Social Groups: Seek out social groups or organizations that align with personal interests and hobbies. This could include book clubs, art classes, cooking groups, or fitness groups. These activities not only provide opportunities for socialization but also allow for the pursuit of personal passions.*

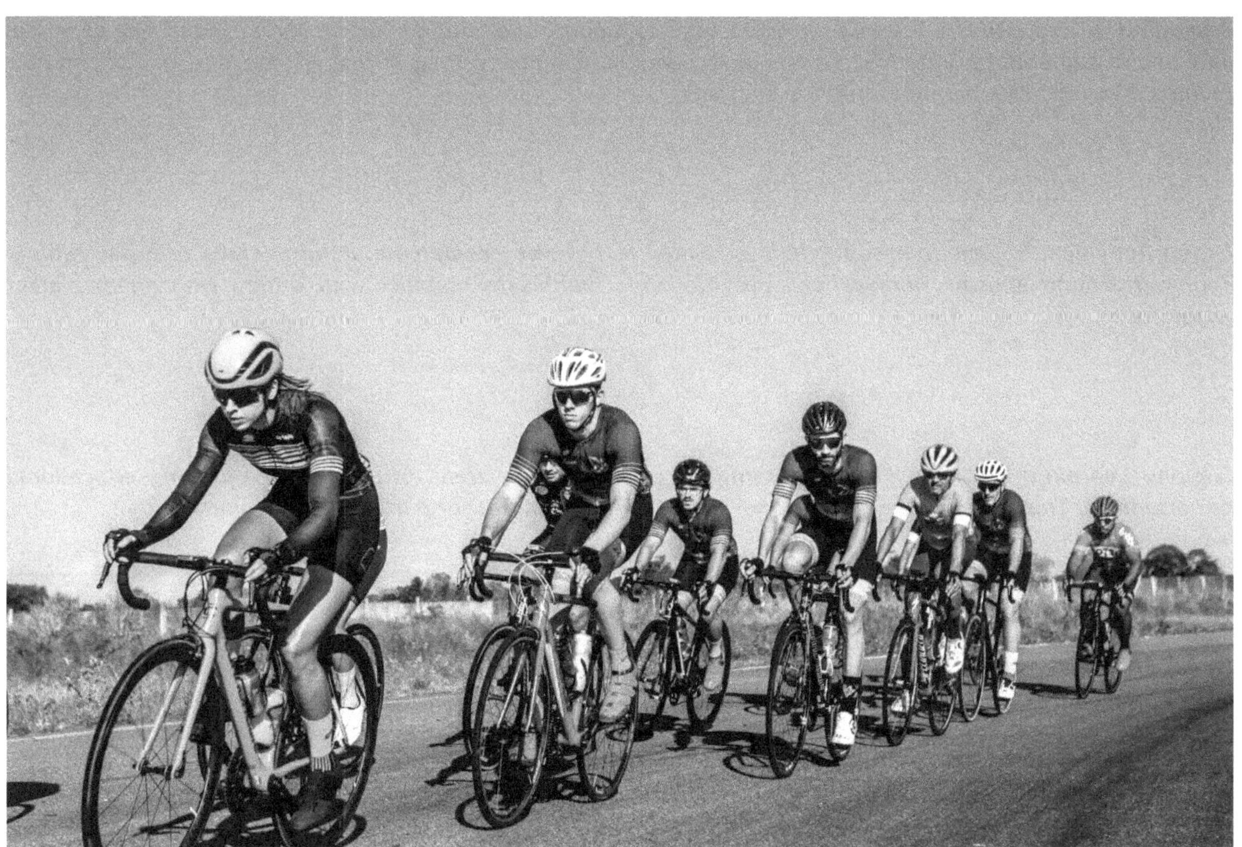

*Technology and Social Media: Embrace technology and social media platforms to connect with friends, family, and communities. Virtual platforms provide a convenient way to stay in touch, join online communities, and engage in group activities, even from the comfort of home.*

### C. Incorporating Hobbies and Interests into Daily Routines

*Incorporating hobbies and interests into daily routines can add fulfillment and enjoyment to life. Engaging in activities that bring personal satisfaction contributes to overall well-being and a sense of purpose. Here are some ways to incorporate hobbies and interests:*

*Set Aside Dedicated Time: Allocate specific time in your schedule for pursuing hobbies and interests. Treat this time as an essential part of your daily routine and prioritize it as you would any other commitment.*

*Integrate Hobbies into Everyday Tasks: Find ways to incorporate hobbies into everyday tasks. For example, listening to audiobooks or podcasts while exercising, painting or crafting during leisure time, or cooking new recipes that align with personal culinary interests.*

*Group Activities: Engage in group activities related to hobbies or interests. Joining clubs or organizations centered around specific hobbies can provide opportunities to connect with others who share similar passions.*

*Lifelong Learning: Embrace lifelong learning by exploring new areas of interest or pursuing educational opportunities. This could include taking courses, attending lectures, or participating in workshops.*

*By promoting an active lifestyle, nurturing social connections, and incorporating hobbies and interests into daily routines, older adults can enhance their overall well-being and maintain a vibrant and fulfilling life.*

# *Conclusion*

*In this book, we have explored the essential aspects of healthy aging and senior fitness, addressing the unique needs of older adults. Throughout the chapters, we have highlighted the importance of mobility, fall prevention, cognitive health, nutrition, social connections, and overcoming barriers to exercise. As we conclude this journey, let's recap the key points and takeaways, encourage embracing healthy aging and senior fitness, and reflect on maintaining overall health and well-being in older adulthood.*

## *A. Recap of Key Points and Takeaways*

*Aging Process and Its Impact: The aging process brings changes to our bodies, including decreased mobility and an increased risk of age-related conditions. Recognizing these changes allows us to address them proactively.*

*Exercise for Healthy Aging: Regular exercise plays a vital role in maintaining mobility, preventing falls, improving cognitive function, and promoting overall well-being. It is never too late to start exercising, and even small steps can make a significant difference.*

*Assessing Individual Needs: Evaluating physical capabilities and limitations, identifying specific health concerns, and tailoring exercise programs to individual needs ensure safety and effectiveness.*

*Nutrition and Healthy Eating Habits: A balanced diet provides the necessary nutrients for healthy aging. Considering nutritional requirements and adopting healthy eating habits contribute to overall well-being.*

*Social Connections and Mental Stimulation: Engaging in social activities, pursuing hobbies, and stimulating the mind help maintain cognitive health and emotional well-being.*

*Overcoming Barriers: Addressing common barriers to exercise, such as physical limitations, lack of confidence, time constraints, and social support, is crucial for maintaining an active lifestyle.*

*Embracing healthy aging and senior fitness is a lifelong journey that brings numerous benefits. It is an opportunity to enhance our quality of life, maintain independence, and enjoy the golden years to the fullest. Regardless of our current fitness level or age, we can make positive changes and strive for better health. Embrace the belief that it is never too late to start, and every step taken towards a healthier lifestyle matters.*

## C. Final Thoughts on Maintaining Overall Health and Well-being in Older Adulthood

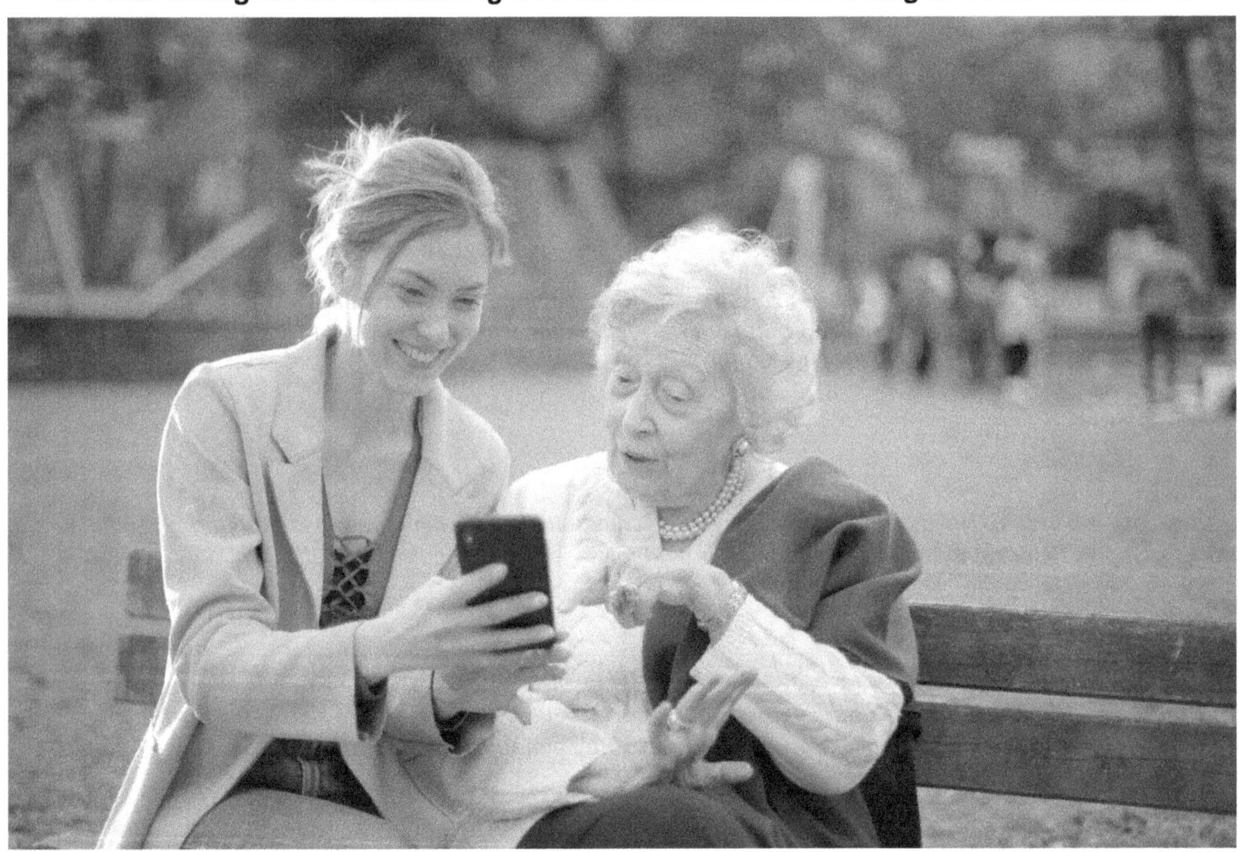

*As we conclude, let us reflect on the importance of maintaining overall health and well-being in older adulthood. Aging is a natural process, and while we cannot control all aspects of it, we can take proactive steps to promote our well-being. By embracing healthy habits, staying physically active, nurturing social connections, nourishing our bodies with nutritious food, and seeking continuous personal growth, we can lead fulfilling lives well into our later years.*

*Remember, healthy aging is not just about the physical aspects but also encompasses emotional, social, and cognitive well-being. It is about finding joy in each day, celebrating achievements, and adapting to change with resilience and grace. Together, let us embark on this journey of healthy aging and senior fitness, empowering ourselves and others to embrace a life of vitality and well-being.*

*Here's to a future of vibrant health and happiness in our journey of healthy aging!*

www.ingramcontent.com/pod-product-compliance
Lightning Source LLC
Chambersburg PA
CBHW081827250726
48657CB00011B/3505